A RUNNER'S DIET

A Comprehensive Guide to Fulfilling your Nutrition Needs for Training and Competition and Weight Loss

Brought to you by:

New Guy Series

A Runner's Diet

A Comprehensive Guide to Fulfilling your Nutrition Needs for Training and Competition

Written By: ***Chris Alexander***

Edited By: **Barry Kephart**

First Printing: 2015

New Guy Series

2850 Oak Road

Pearland, Tx 77584

www.newguyseries.com

Disclaimer

The medical and/or nutritional information in this eBook is not intended to be a substitute for professional medical advice, diagnosis, or treatment. Always seek the advice of your physician or other qualified health provider with any questions you may have regarding a medical condition. Never disregard professional medical advice or delay seeking it because of something you have read in this eBook.

Contents

Introduction

On Your Mark, Get Set, Eat!

You may have the best fitness, but there is still something that can stand between you and your success as a runner: **Wrong education about nutrient intake!**

There is a lot of wrong information circulating around about runner's nutrition on the internet, which has given rise to various misconceptions that affect the very form and performance of athletes.

These are the issues we seek to address in this eBook.

Why Make the Effort?

It needs to be explained why we bothered to assemble such a document and why you should devote some time to go through it.

You see, distance running is getting more popular by the day. Statistics from the past couple of years show that more and more runners are trying to achieve the 26.2 mile landmark, and that more than 450,000 (and counting) American runners have successfully finished marathons.

This is not just another fitness fad. Running is a time-honored test of strength, endurance, stamina, and of course, proper hydration and nutrition. Modern runners are following in the footsteps of the soldier

Pheidippides in ancient Greece, who at the close of the 5th century BC ran from Marathon to Athens, and legend has it that he died upon reaching his destination.

Who knows? Maybe he didn't eat right...

Why Study About Nutrition?

Now as the mileage of the average runner is increasing, so is his/her calorie needs. This especially includes calories derived from carbohydrates.

To perform optimally, runners require anywhere from 7 to 10g of carbohydrate/kg of body weight while they train. And when running long distance, they should strive to keep the carbohydrate count to as close to 10g/kg as possible.

This carbohydrate intake will help their bodies saturate the muscles with Glycogen, which is necessary for endurance training. Hence, carbohydrates should form up to 65% of a runner's diet. During daily training, it can be 55% as well.

You may say, *'I already know what my nutrition needs are'*. It's good that you do. But do you know how to fulfill these needs? Are you consuming all the wrong sources of nutrition? Many runners do.

To reiterate the previous point, running cannot be done right without a mindful approach. Everything you eat and drink has a direct impact on your track performance.

Why take the chance?

Follow the guidelines presented in this eBook and tweak your running nutrition in a way that every calorie you consume takes you the distance.

Chapter 1

Runners CANNOT Eat Everything They Like

'I'm not running the Olympics, and besides I run for 90 minutes a day. Why should I even bother about by diet? That much running will burn anything, right?'

Wrong.

Before we start discussing nutrition for runners, it is vital to deal with the myth that runners can eat anything as long as they are working out enough.

In his book 'The Last Pick' athlete and philanthropist Dave McGillivray (race director of the Boston Marathon) revealed how he also adhered to this myth. To quote the man *'if the furnace was hot enough, it would burn everything'*

However, at the age of 57, he was diagnosed with coronary artery disease in 2013, much to his own surprise.

Even doctors have lent credence, in the past, to the idea that since running for miles on end keeps weight, blood pressure, heart rate, and cholesterol levels in check, and thereby give license to athletes to eat as they please. This way of thinking is being set aside for a smarter approach to the nutritional needs of athletes.

However, recent research shows otherwise. The study in question (published in the current edition of Missouri Medicine) took 50 volunteers who had run at least one marathon in the last 2.5 decades and compared their health with a control group.

What was discovered is surprising: The 50 men who were active runners had higher levels of coronary-artery plaque than the control group comprised of men who led a sedentary lifestyle.

Another study from last year (published in the British Medical Journal) compared the carotid arteries of 42 volunteers (runners who had qualified for the Boston Marathon) with their less active spouses. The assumption behind the study was that the runners would have a better atherosclerotic risk profile, but the results showed otherwise.

There is another line of research that is seeking to establish that extreme-endurance exercise can actually give rise of heart problems instead of preventing or treating them. Some cardiologists are adopting the theory that after a certain point, heavy workouts can actually cause heart disease instead of preventing it. Conditions include coronary artery disease, myocardial fibrosis, and even sudden cardiac death.

And while there may not be conclusive evidence to establish this link, the reports of heart disease in runners are increasing by the day.

But our concerns are not to do with the extremity of the workout (which is beyond the scope of this presentation), but more with the Runner's Diet. In this respect, all experts are unanimous that a high-calorie workout doesn't mean that you eat without discernment.

For these reasons, you need to learn about proper nutrition that ensures your long-term health and success as a runner.

Chapter 2

Snacking Up

Your training plan may have an allotted time for breakfast and dinner (more on this in the next section), your stomach might not stick to schedule. It may grumble during or after the training.

The best way to successfully go through your workout without feeling like you have fasted for 40 days, is to snack up before you run!

Not only will this help you deal with premature fatigue while running, but your blood-sugar levels will also be in check. And when your belly is healthily and comfortable, you also stay motivated to finish the workout.

And don't worry if you are running to lose weight, as there are plenty of healthy snacks that you can munch on pre-workout without loading up on bad calories. Any snack you consume should have carbohydrates for a quick energy boost, electrolytes for maintaining the balance of fluids in the body, and of course protein to suppress hunger. However, avoid fiber and too much fat, even if you are running for an hour, for these can be difficult to digest.

And the best thing about snacks is they are quick to prepare (or sometimes require no preparation at all), which means they will not interfere with your workout schedule.

The following is a list of snacks that you can have before running. We will notify which item is best for varying durations of your workout.

Fruits

Fruits are a great source of nutrients, they provide great taste, and also serve as quick bites requiring no preparation at all. Oranges are a great option in this regard. Not only do they provide nearly all of your daily vitamin C needs, but they also have other benefits apart from providing you energy. For instance, they can help prevent muscle injuries, while also replacing collagen in muscle fibers that break down during exercise. And considering that one orange has just a little more than 60 calories, they are great snack options if you are watching your weight.

Just remember 2 things:

1. A fruit snack like an orange is apt for a 15-30 minute workout run instead of a 30-60 minute workout. But this is not a rule; you just have to see what works for you

2. You have to *eat* the fruits. It is debatable whether juicing provides the same health benefits, as eating that piece of fruit, or not, and the fruit juices available on the market contain sugar, which cannot only increase your carbohydrate intake unnecessarily, but also may upset your stomach. The same holds true for fruits. You can prepare them in a shake or smoothie, but you may have to be creative to

make them as nutritiously viable for a great power snack!

The next set of snacks is meant for 30 to 60 minutes:

Coffee

Wow! Is there something that coffee can't do?

Get any cool coffee beverages like an iced latte or a Frappuccino (no whip cream) which keeps you hydrated while working out in hot climate. Not to mention, the milk can provide you some protein.

The added benefits of having iced coffee drinks is that not only does coffee keep you focused during the run, but it has also been shown to delay muscle fatigue during intense workouts.

Low-Fiber Cereal

High-fiber cereals may be healthy, but they can upset your stomach during a run. It is so much easier for your muscles to convert carbs into energy as compared to fiber-rich foods, so go for cereals with fewer than 2g of fiber per serving. You can eat it plain or with milk. You can also combine it with fruits by topping half a cup of sliced bananas and strawberries on your cereal.

Dried Fruit

When it comes to dried fruit, there is a wide variety that you can try, such as apricots, mangoes, cranberries, and dates. These not only serve as concentrated sources of instant carbohydrates, but also aid in muscle function due to the presence of potassium. Having a few dates is enough to provide you with carbs and potassium, in case you don't like eating a banana!

Note: Dried fruit has more calories than fresh fruit, so avoid eating them like a bag of chips.

Instant Oatmeal

In case you run for more than 60 minutes, instant oatmeal is a great source of whole grains. One pack supplies almost half of your daily iron. You can go ahead and have sweetened instant oatmeal, for the sugar will provide you the energy for longer runs.

Vegetables

Veggies are great, even when you are running for longer durations (60 to 90 minutes).

You should try sweet potatoes that are high in carbs, thereby giving you lasting energy for longer runs. Think of double the daily of intake of vitamin A, sweet potatoes boost up your immune system immensely. The skin of the vegetable is actually soluble fiber, which means pairing it with physical exercise will actually help you shed belly fat. However, if you are having the skin, then eat it at least an hour before you work out. This allows for proper digestion.

Carrots and Hummus

Carrots plus hummus brings a great blend of carbs and protein to your runner's diet, snacks that will keep you full during longer runs. Carrots are not only rich in beta carotene, but there is research to show that eating them can also help prevent skin damage.

Add these benefits with hummus, which contains sodium that makes you want to drink more water.

But in case you like carrots on their own merit, you can always try other snacks with hummus, such as wheat crackers. This combination is filling and also packs an abundance of protein, fiber, vitamin B6, and folic acid.

How Early Before the Run Should You Eat Anything

It's all about the timing. In order to train well and stay healthy, you have to find out how long before the run should you eat. The words 'find out' have been used because there is no one uniform answer to how early before a run should you eat. This is something that varies from runner to runner. While some can get started after 10-15 minutes of snacking up, others may require longer for their system to properly digest, sometimes 1-2 hours. Hence, you will have to do some testing to determine which time is right for you.

Note that some runners will tell you that they have no issues in eating and running. Some sort of eating is necessary, because running on an empty stomach can leave you out of energy and severely fatigued.

So what you need to do with your training and eating is to know, from your own experiences, just how much you are able to eat before a run.

A rule of thumb is that you eat a snack or light meal *at least* an hour before you start running. If you are having a heavy meal, then ideally you should give 3 to 4 hours for digestion.

Of course, this shouldn't be a problem for those that are running in a "fast mode" (more on this later). But the fasting mode doesn't work for every runner, and even then it is only suited for moderate, 30 minute runs. If this is the duration of your workout, then you can manage with water along with a sports drink or energy gel.

But for longer and more intense running sessions, you need to saddle up with 300-500 calories before hitting the tracks. Determine how much you can eat to have a trouble-free run, and there is no choice but to eat at this time. If you like to run early in the morning, then now you have to wake up even earlier.

Avoiding Stomach Problems

Along with the right timing, it is also necessary that you eat the right kind of foods before the run so that you don't feel the urge to find a bathroom during the workout or race. Go for something that is high in carbohydrates but low in protein, fiber, and fat.

Here are some helpful suggestions in this regard:

- Bagel with peanut butter
- Turkey and cheese with bread
- Bananas
- Energy bars
- Cold cereal with milk
- Whole wheat toast with peanut butter
- Applesauce
- Low fat Yogurt

Note that while caffeine has been recommended in this eBook time and again, coffee and other caffeinated beverages can cause gastro-intestinal distress. Once again, you need to ascertain what works for you. This may take a trial and error approach, but once you figure out how your body likes to be fueled for optimum performance, you will be happy that you took the time.

Chapter 3

What to Eat During the Run

As much as it is important what you eat before and after your runs, you have to ensure that your energy levels stay up during the run as well. This applies to both professional athletes and fitness enthusiasts.

Eating during a run may not be the oldest concept in the corpus of athlete nutrition. So of course you may not find it easy to adopt this habit.

Consider this also a part of your trial eating. It is better to get started with eating during the training when you go for longer runs. This is because the longer runs will allow your stomach to digest carbohydrates while you are in motion.

But when you are experimenting with eating during running, stick to tried and tested foods.

Why Eat While Running?

To understand this, you need to know how long on average can a person run without requiring refueling. Usually, any running workout under 1 hour can be done without refueling, provided that you had a proper pre-workout meal or snack.

If you plan to run over 60 minutes, you should consider consuming small amounts of high-GI (glycemic index) carbohydrates. This will help you maintain a good pace of running as your working muscles get re-fueled. In addition, your blood Glucose levels will also remain in balance.

As the body absorbs these carbohydrates, your brain will also be fuelled, which allows you to retain your focus and motivation during the run. The psychological impetus will come in handy especially when your muscles begin to wear out.

Wouldn't I Feel Full?

Running on a full stomach is something that most runners avoid. Some suggest that you should never run immediately after consuming more than 200-300 calories.

So, if you just had a 'heavy meal' (containing several ounces of protein or meat, vegetables, and carbohydrates), ideally you should wait for at least 3 hours before running to allow for proper digestion.

The heavier the meal, the greater the energy required to digest it. The body directs more blood flow to the stomach and other internal organs to facilitate this process (now you wonder why you feel sleepy after lunch).

So since the blood flow is directed to the belly, there is less available blood flow for the legs and arms in a quantity fit for endurance training. The opposite happens when you run; the blood flow is now directed towards the large working muscles to provide the necessary energy for muscle contraction.

That is why with a large amount of food in your stomach, running can be difficult, sometimes impossible. Our bodies are not designed in a way to help us run long distances and digest large amounts of food at the same time. Mixing the two functions can cause a host of problems including but not restricted to:

- Stomach cramps
- Stomach aches
- Gastro-intestinal distress

However, we are not telling you to have a 3-course meal before or during your run. When training, stick to high-GI carbohydrate options that can be absorbed easily. This will help you prevent nausea or any other form of discomfort during a run.

When to Eat During the Run

Feeling hungry should not be seen as a signal for refueling during the run. Like most things described in this book, you will have to discover your refueling needs by trial and error and find a strategy you are comfortable with. What works most often is taking in carbohydrates in small quantities, but with great frequency. See how this strategy works for you.

On average, a marathon runner can take 30-60g of carbs per hour which keeps him/her moving. Food items in this regard include cereal bars, energy bar, jellied sweets, and large bananas.

Note that fluids work best during runs, but these will be covered in a later chapter.

Chapter 4

Post-Run Eating

Skipping proper meals after a run can lead to lethargy and sugar cravings. But these are only the immediate consequences. In the long-run, skipping post-run meals can lead to both sickness and injuries.

You can put off not eating anything for 30-60 minutes after your run, but it is vital to have a snack or full meal within an hour or two. But don't push yourself; eat something within 30 minutes post-workout as your body requires the essential nutrients to assist both muscle growth and repair.

As in pre-workout meals, both proteins and carbohydrates are equally essential for post-workout recovery. Being the main source of fuel for the body, carbohydrates are stored as Glycogen in the muscles and liver. But there is only so much that your body can store. The same is true for protein.

This is why you need to refill your fuel tank before it is empty to not only continue running without burning out, but also preventing serious tissue injury.

As far as protein intake is concerned, 20g is sufficient to kick start and power the recovery process after running. Any regular 500ml milkshake will cater to your needs. You can also consider having a sandwich with lean meats, eggs, or low-fat cheese.

Yogurt is also a great option. You can have Greek yogurt, granola and mixed berries. A fruit smoothie made of natural yogurt is also a great choice.

"What if I Am Watching My Weight"?

You need to balance recovery with weight loss after a run. This will take some experimenting to get right. As a general rule, you have to adjust your daily carbohydrate intake proportionate to your training. So intake needs to be higher on days where you increase the time and/or intensity of the run and vice-versa.

A helpful tip for those that are managing their weight is to have low-GI carbohydrate foods at meal time instead of consuming a lot of high-GI snacks. Also try to have proper meals instead of recovery snacks following a workout. Of course, this will require more planning on your part as you combine runs with mealtimes, but eating meals instead of snacks boost your energy more. Since you are reducing the overall amount of caloric intake, since you aren't eating all the extra snacks after a workout and before the meal, this will help with reducing overall weight.

Here is a list of foods that are good for recovery:

- Oatmeal

While all foods we recommend offer carbohydrates and protein, oatmeal also contains fiber as well. This makes you feel full, which avoids over-indulgence (which can be a powerful temptation after a race or a heavy workout). And if you don't like the bland taste, you can always add a fruit topping to boost both taste and health.

- Hummus

Can you tell that we love Hummus?

- Chicken Breasts

Chicken breasts are filled with protein. But while runners can have them at any time of the day, what especially makes them apt for a post-workout meal is that they are easy to prepare. Add in microwavable steamed rice (preferably brown rice) and frozen vegetables, and you have a well-rounded meal on your table within minutes.

- Salmon

Salmon not only contains omega-3 fatty acids, but antioxidants as well. The latter work with your immune system to fight against free radicals. And the best part is that you can get pre-cooked salmon as well. Just heat and serve.

- Almonds

Almonds also provide antioxidants and fiber, and if consumed regularly, they can even lower cholesterol. The best part is that there is no one way of eating them. For example, you can have almonds alone or you can mix them with a yogurt or a fruit drink. Sliced almonds can also be featured on your pasta or salad.

Here are some additional suggestions:

- Cottage Cheese
- Greek Yogurt with mixed berries
- Chocolate Milk
- Banana with peanut butter (or almond butter)
- Protein bar (check the label)
- Turkey sandwich on whole wheat bread (hummus, or light mayo for healthy fat).

Chapter 5

Creating a Plan

We can list all the possible meals that are healthy for runners, but that would only double (nay triple) the size of this eBook. Not to mention, it's not only important to know what to eat but also when to eat it. Hence, in this section, you will learn how to develop a nutrition plan.

Why Develop a Plan?

You may have a foundational knowledge of what constitutes a runner's diet, but even then you are better off creating a plan. Plans bring order and discipline into your life, things that are essential for developing health and fitness. Note that what we are talking about here are plans created on paper or any digital format (instead of the inside your head) where you can check them from time to time.

One of the greatest benefits of creating a plan is that you will eat out less. Now athletes are not prohibited from eat out, and an increasing number of restaurants are offering healthier items on their menus, especially to accommodate customers with Gluten intolerance, food allergies, and other dietary issues.

The same holds true for prepackaged meals. When you have a workable plan in close range, you will be sure to get all the right groceries and make that your stock never goes empty. Other benefits include:

- By being more mindful of what you eat, you will naturally waste fewer groceries. Many people bring items like broccoli and lettuce thinking that they will eat them, but the veggies end up at a corner of the kitchen looking like a science experiment. Not to mention, this also translates to fewer trips to the grocery store.

- This also means that you will have less processed foods in your diet and more healthy ones. Remember what you learned in an earlier section: even if you are running 3 miles or more every day, you can't simply eat anything that comes your way.

- The choice of meals increases when you are following a nutrition plan and eating healthy. Just look at all the nutritious meals and snacks we have listed in this eBook, and there are many more than you can find online and in cookbooks. Not to mention, when you have a basic idea of how much carbs and protein your body needs at a given time, you can always improvise!

- You will never be confused as to what to eat (for some people, choosing what to eat is as stressful as a choosing a career!) What you need for each day of the week will be listed on the fridge (or wherever you have put up your list)

- You are never caught off guard on busy days as regards to what you should eat, so even the most hectic schedule doesn't allow you to indulge in fast food

- With a proper nutrition plan in place, you will avoid the stress of needlessly looking inside the fridge and wondering what you should make today

- Your nutrition plan will be tailored to meet the individual needs of your body, which means you can work around allergies, intolerance, and other dietary issues that can interfere with your workouts

- Another byproduct that many athletes notice of planning out meals and acting on that plan is that their healthy diet becomes a very healthy diet! The more often you eat healthy and what your body really needs, the less you will have those nagging french fry and double bacon cheese burger cravings.

Last but not least, there is a financial side to creating food plans as well. One of the ways in which this materializes itself is that you are eating out on fewer occasions. And when you make a visit to grocery, you will not be driven in making impulsive purchases since you very well know what you have to eat.

How to Create a Nutrition Plan

Creating a nutrition plan is an essential component of your runner's fitness since nutrition can both maximize performance or adversely affect it.

When you are training as a runner, the calories you consume in one day should reflect the total volume of training. In sports terminology, this is known as 'periodizing' in training. This is necessary not only for improving performance, but also to reduce the risk of injury.

When you over-train or do not follow the proper running techniques, you will end up hurting yourself instead of boosting endurance.

Hence, depending on how much you train in one day, your nutrition plan for training should at least be divided into three sections.

Here is a sample training plan. We are making the assumption that you run on alternative days of the week with varying intensities.

So for instance:

- You rest on Monday,
- followed by a moderate run of 30-45 minutes on Tuesday
- Rest on Wednesday
- An increase an intensity on Thursday (60-90 minutes)

- Moderate exercise on Friday
- Rest on Saturday
- Intensive work out on Sunday

Here's how you can further divide your nutrition plan:

Eating on Days of Rest

To start off, since you are not training, you should lower your carb-intake. So if you are having a carbohydrate-based breakfast or lunch, that is more than enough. Instead, have more protein, preferably in your breakfast which will keep you full until lunch time.

Why protein? Because it helps the development of muscle tissue and also repairs damage, especially if you had an intense workout the day before.

To further aid the recovery process, you should also increase consumption of polyunsaturated fats. These also help to reduce inflammation. In addition, since running produces free radicals, you should consume fruits and vegetables that are rich in antioxidants to combat them. Fruits and veggies can also help reduce muscle soreness following training.

Finally, on rest days, you can think about trying out new recipes and condiments.

Suggestions

Breakfast

- Scrambled eggs
- Bran flakes cereal/low fat milk

- Cottage cheese with mixed fruit
- Western style omelet

Lunch

- Boca burgers with fruit
- Chicken fajita (can add tomato, lettuce, and onion)
- Turkey club wrap
- Chicken salad wrap
- Tuna wrap

Dinner

- Chicken and brown rice
- Turkey burger (lean)
- Salmon with red potatoes and vegetable
- Ground turkey, Rice, and Broccoli stir-fry

Note: If you feel hungry through the day, you can always have light snacks like a turkey roll up (low sodium), Edamame, or sting cheese, and fruit.

Eating on Moderate Workout Days

Most of the guidelines mentioned above are applicable for moderate workout days as well. However, you should consider running in a 'fasting' state, that is, running for 30-45 minutes in a low to moderate intensity mode should be done before breakfast.

The logic is that when muscles aren't properly 'fuelled' before the workout session, they come under stress, and in this state, they adapt and become more efficient. In addition, the body breaks down fat and uses it fuel for training, thereby helping you lose weight.

However, you may not find it easy to adapt to the fasting-running method. In any case, you should never employ this strategy for high-intensity training sessions.

Training Sessions 60 minutes or Above-Moderate Training

Training sessions over 60 minutes can be further divided into two more categories:

- Moderate intensity or moderate intensity with high intensity intervals
- High intensity training or more than 1 training session per day

In this section, we deal with the former.

To start off, you should go for moderate intake of carbohydrates. Including carbs in your breakfast and lunch not only help you during training but also assist in refilling your Glycogen reserves. You can reduce the carbohydrate intake at dinner.

The same holds true for protein intake as well. Have a small serving protein should be included in each meal.

Moving on, add polyunsaturated fats in your evening meal to boost muscle cell function.

But most importantly, make sure that all your meals on these days include foods containing iron. This is necessary to provide oxygen to the working muscles and also to assist in energy production as you engage in endurance exercise.

Suggestions

Breakfast

- Scrambled Egg Muffin
- Honey crunch granola with apricots and almonds
- Bran flakes cereal with protein powder

Lunch

- Cranberry pecan chicken salad wrap
- Tuna Salad with Side of Fruit
- Chicken Fajita

Dinner

- Shrimp, Rice, and Vegetable Stir-Fry
- Smoked mackerel
- Pork tenderloin with asparagus

Note: Have salads with these dinner options (Smoked mackerel with orange & couscous salad, Tamborine chicken with summer vegetable bowl, and Teriyaki tuna skewers with Butternut squash salad)

The dinner options have been focused on low-GI carbs. So if you choose to try dinner options other than the three listed above, make sure they include low-GI carbohydrates for sustained energy release.

And if you feel hungry between meals, you can go for snacks like apricot, honey on Whole Wheat toast, and pistachio Protein bar, Turkey and avocado toast (in the afternoon), and melon and crunchy bran pots in the evening.

Training Sessions 60 minutes or Above-Intensive Training

The following is the nutrition plan for heavy training days where you either have a long intensive session, or have more than one training sessions.

On these days, you have to increase your carbohydrate intake, with a serving of carbs featured in every meal of the day. These are also the days where you should snack up between meals, especially high-GI carbohydrate snacks before you start training.

Start the day off with a low-GI breakfast to provide you enough energy for the earlier part of the day and your run. You should have more carbs to limit fat.

Have your protein after the workouts, preferably as part of the evening snack. Great ideas include creamy mango and coconut smoothie, or spiced hot chocolate. These will help your body to recover from the heavy training and also to support muscle growth during the night. Be sure to mix in your protein though. You won't see any increase in fitness if you walk around drinking hot chocolate all day.

Another important thing to remember is that you need to pay close attention to is your fluid intake. You need to keep yourself hydrated for sweat losses during the training.

Suggestions

<u>Breakfast</u>

- Bran Flakes with Protein Powder
- Cinnamon buckwheat pancakes with cherries
- Cottage Cheese with Fruit and Nuts (great snack also)

<u>Lunch Options</u>

- Quick chili bean wraps
- Falafel burgers
- Chicken and broccoli pasta bake

<u>Dinner</u>

- Lamb with buckwheat noodles
- Chicken, sweet potato
- Spanish rice and Chicken
- Salmon with Red Potatoes

Since you need to have snacks as well, here are some helpful options:

<u>Morning</u>

- Banana with Greek Yogurt
- Banana and blueberry muffins
- Cinnamon berry granola bars

Afternoon

- Instant frozen berry yogurt

Note: Earlier in the book we discussed how you should experiment with your eating habits to see how early before the run should you eat. An additional tip is that you should never try out new meals and snacks on intensive workout days. Especially avoid foods that are known to cause gastrointestinal issues. This also applies to a "race day". Nothing new should be tried out at the last second. Once you have learned what works for you, use it and tweak it. Varying greatly from a plan that works very well for can lead to all sorts of uncomfortable situations.

Chapter 6

Supplements

Ideally, athletes should get all their nutrient needs from whole foods, which is no impossible feat. Couple this with the fact that there is no string evidence that supports the assertion that taking supplements can enhance runner performance.

However, some runners out there may have nutrient deficiencies which may be affecting their performance. Iron deficiency, for instance, can lead to severe feedback.

Once again, which any such deficiency can be catered with proper diet, a doctor may recommend supplements. And this is our advice to you: only take supplements on your doctor's recommendation.

You can of course take supplements that you have found assist in keeping the correct and healthy levels of a certain vitamin or mineral. But you shouldn't need to pop 5 pills first thing in the morning to keep those levels where they need to be.

Chapter 7

Hydration

In the last section of this eBook, we will talk a little about hydration. Whether you are an athlete or someone who has adopted running as an exercise, proper hydration is of critical importance. Proper intake of fluids is not only important for recovering water leaving the body as sweat, but also to regulate body temperature, keeping joints lubricating, and transporting nutrients for energy.

And while water is enough for the body's hydration needs, sports drink are also helpful, especially if you are running at a high intensity for more than an hour. Sports drinks contain calories, potassium, and other essential nutrients to provide the body with energy and electrolytes to help you performing optimally for longer time periods.

However, you need to be discerning when it comes to sports drinks, as most of the brands available on the market are high in calories, sugar, and sodium. Also be careful of the serving size. One bottle contains several servings, so make sure that you multiply the information on the Nutrition Facts Label by 2 or 3, depending on the information on that bottle's label. Also remember that if your sports drink contains caffeine, you should reduce caffeine intake from other sources.

Hydration Before a Run

If you are approaching a long run or race, you need to stay well-hydrated not only immediately before the event, but for a few days leading up to the run. A simple of checking if you are properly hydrated is having large volumes of pale urine at least 6 times a day.

Abstain from alcohol before a run, as it dehydrates you and can also get in the way of getting proper rest.

When it's one hour before the run, try to drink 16 ounces of water or a sports drink. And just like your pre-workout meals, you need to experiment during training how much can you drink before a run to avoid the urge to urinate.

Drinking During the Run

A 2010 study shows that using a carbohydrate-based sports drink as a mouth rinse can help to activate the brain and lower fatigue during a run. So, you should include carbohydrate-electrolyte sports drinks to meet your fuel and fluid needs.

Caffeine-based drinks are also helpful in this regard, especially in the later part of the training session or race. Many sports drinks available on the market do contain caffeine.

Note that when it comes to fulfilling the 30g carbohydrate requirement during the run, drinks fare better than solid foods. Fluids are also helpful for those who cannot eat immediately after a run.

Post-run Hydration

There's no question about it; you should begin to rehydrate with a bottle of water or sports drink immediately after your run. This is not time to gulp. But a few sips every minute or so will get the fluids in and begin to get you hydrated. For every pound lost, you need to drink at least 20 fl oz. And if you see that your urine is dark yellow after the run, this is a sign that you need more rehydration.

This is another point that you will need to learn based on your own body. Some people require more or less constant hydration during a workout without "feeling" like they are thirsty. A good rule of thumb is that you should drink and eat before you feel thirsty or hungry. This will ensure that you maintain your hydration and caloric needs throughout the exercise. This doesn't mean to chug water and sports drinks the entire time, moderation is still key here. Just don't wait till your mouth is bone dry before getting a drink!

Conclusion

That's about it!

Remember that reaching your full athletic potential heavily relies on proper sports nutrition. And to that end, we have tried to cover the various aspects of the runner's diet in this brief presentation.

However, as we have repeated time and again, the physical needs of each runner are unique. Hence, we encourage you to not only use the generalized information of this book for your benefit, but also stay in close contact with your doctor and if possible, a sports nutritionist as well.

Good luck and Happy Running!